December

Week 1

12/31/18 to 01/06/19

○ 31. MONDAY

DINNER PLANS

○ 1. TUESDAY

○ 2. WEDNESDAY

TO DO

○ 3. THURSDAY

○ 4. FRIDAY

○ 5. SATURDAY / 6. SUNDAY

January

Week 2

01/07/19 to 01/13/19

○ 7. MONDAY

DINNER PLANS

○ 8. TUESDAY

○ 9. WEDNESDAY

TO DO

○ 10. THURSDAY

○ 11. FRIDAY

○ 12. SATURDAY / 13. SUNDAY

January

Week 3

01/14/19 to 01/20/19

○ 14. MONDAY

DINNER PLANS

○ 15. TUESDAY

○ 16. WEDNESDAY

TO DO

○ 17. THURSDAY

○ 18. FRIDAY

○ 19. SATURDAY / 20. SUNDAY

January

Week 4

01/21/19 to 01/27/19

○ 21. MONDAY

DINNER PLANS

○ 22. TUESDAY

○ 23. WEDNESDAY

TO DO

○ 24. THURSDAY

○ 25. FRIDAY

○ 26. SATURDAY / 27. SUNDAY

January

Week 5

01/28/19 to 02/03/19

○ 28. MONDAY

DINNER PLANS

○ 29. TUESDAY

○ 30. WEDNESDAY

TO DO

○ 31. THURSDAY

○ 1. FRIDAY

○ 2. SATURDAY / 3. SUNDAY

February

Week 6   02/04/19 to 02/10/19

○ 4. MONDAY

                                                DINNER PLANS

○ 5. TUESDAY

○ 6. WEDNESDAY

                                                TO DO

○ 7. THURSDAY

○ 8. FRIDAY

○ 9. SATURDAY / 10. SUNDAY

February

○ 11. MONDAY

DINNER PLANS

○ 12. TUESDAY

○ 13. WEDNESDAY

TO DO

○ 14. THURSDAY

○ 15. FRIDAY

○ 16. SATURDAY / 17. SUNDAY

February

Week 8

02/18/19 to 02/24/19

○ 18. MONDAY

DINNER PLANS

○ 19. TUESDAY

○ 20. WEDNESDAY

TO DO

○ 21. THURSDAY

○ 22. FRIDAY

○ 23. SATURDAY / 24. SUNDAY

February

Week 9

02/25/19 to 03/03/19

○ 25. MONDAY

DINNER PLANS

○ 26. TUESDAY

○ 27. WEDNESDAY

TO DO

○ 28. THURSDAY

○ 1. FRIDAY

○ 2. SATURDAY / 3. SUNDAY

March

Week 10   03/04/19 to 03/10/19

○ 4. MONDAY

DINNER PLANS

○ 5. TUESDAY

○ 6. WEDNESDAY

TO DO

○ 7. THURSDAY

○ 8. FRIDAY

○ 9. SATURDAY / 10. SUNDAY

March

Week 11

03/11/19 to 03/17/19

○ 11. MONDAY

DINNER PLANS

○ 12. TUESDAY

○ 13. WEDNESDAY

TO DO

○ 14. THURSDAY

○ 15. FRIDAY

○ 16. SATURDAY / 17. SUNDAY

March

Week 12   03/18/19 to 03/24/19

○ 18. MONDAY

DINNER PLANS

○ 19. TUESDAY

○ 20. WEDNESDAY

TO DO

○ 21. THURSDAY

○ 22. FRIDAY

○ 23. SATURDAY / 24. SUNDAY

March

Week 13   03/25/19 to 03/31/19

○ 25. MONDAY

DINNER PLANS

○ 26. TUESDAY

○ 27. WEDNESDAY

TO DO

○ 28. THURSDAY

○ 29. FRIDAY

○ 30. SATURDAY / 31. SUNDAY

April

04/01/19 to 04/07/19

○ 1. MONDAY

DINNER PLANS

○ 2. TUESDAY

○ 3. WEDNESDAY

TO DO

○ 4. THURSDAY

○ 5. FRIDAY

○ 6. SATURDAY / 7. SUNDAY

April

Week 15

04/08/19 to 04/14/19

○ 8. MONDAY

DINNER PLANS

○ 9. TUESDAY

○ 10. WEDNESDAY

TO DO

○ 11. THURSDAY

○ 12. FRIDAY

○ 13. SATURDAY / 14. SUNDAY

April

Week 16

04/15/19 to 04/21/19

○ 15. MONDAY

DINNER PLANS

○ 16. TUESDAY

○ 17. WEDNESDAY

TO DO

○ 18. THURSDAY

○ 19. FRIDAY

○ 20. SATURDAY / 21. SUNDAY

April

Week 17

04/22/19 to 04/28/19

○ 22. MONDAY

DINNER PLANS

○ 23. TUESDAY

○ 24. WEDNESDAY

TO DO

○ 25. THURSDAY

○ 26. FRIDAY

○ 27. SATURDAY / 28. SUNDAY

April

Week 18

04/29/19 to 05/05/19

○ 29. MONDAY

DINNER PLANS

○ 30. TUESDAY

○ 1. WEDNESDAY

TO DO

○ 2. THURSDAY

○ 3. FRIDAY

○ 4. SATURDAY / 5. SUNDAY

May

Week 19

05/06/19 to 05/12/19

○ 6. MONDAY

DINNER PLANS

○ 7. TUESDAY

○ 8. WEDNESDAY

TO DO

○ 9. THURSDAY

○ 10. FRIDAY

○ 11. SATURDAY / 12. SUNDAY

May

Week 20

05/13/19 to 05/19/19

○ 13. MONDAY

DINNER PLANS

○ 14. TUESDAY

○ 15. WEDNESDAY

TO DO

○ 16. THURSDAY

○ 17. FRIDAY

○ 18. SATURDAY / 19. SUNDAY

May

05/20/19 to 05/26/19

○ 20. MONDAY

DINNER PLANS

○ 21. TUESDAY

○ 22. WEDNESDAY

TO DO

○ 23. THURSDAY

○ 24. FRIDAY

○ 25. SATURDAY / 26. SUNDAY

May

Week 22

05/27/19 to 06/02/19

O 27. MONDAY

DINNER PLANS

O 28. TUESDAY

O 29. WEDNESDAY

TO DO

O 30. THURSDAY

O 31. FRIDAY

O 1. SATURDAY / 2. SUNDAY

June

Week 23

06/03/19 to 06/09/19

○ 3. MONDAY

DINNER PLANS

○ 4. TUESDAY

○ 5. WEDNESDAY

TO DO

○ 6. THURSDAY

○ 7. FRIDAY

○ 8. SATURDAY / 9. SUNDAY

June

Week 24

06/10/19 to 06/16/19

○ 10. MONDAY

DINNER PLANS

○ 11. TUESDAY

○ 12. WEDNESDAY

TO DO

○ 13. THURSDAY

○ 14. FRIDAY

○ 15. SATURDAY / 16. SUNDAY

June

Week 25

06/17/19 to 06/23/19

○ 17. MONDAY

DINNER PLANS

○ 18. TUESDAY

○ 19. WEDNESDAY

TO DO

○ 20. THURSDAY

○ 21. FRIDAY

○ 22. SATURDAY / 23. SUNDAY

June

Week 26

06/24/19 to 06/30/19

○ 24. MONDAY

DINNER PLANS

○ 25. TUESDAY

○ 26. WEDNESDAY

TO DO

○ 27. THURSDAY

○ 28. FRIDAY

○ 29. SATURDAY / 30. SUNDAY

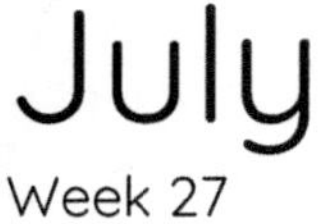

July

Week 27

07/01/19 to 07/07/19

○ 1. MONDAY

DINNER PLANS

○ 2. TUESDAY

○ 3. WEDNESDAY

TO DO

○ 4. THURSDAY

○ 5. FRIDAY

○ 6. SATURDAY / 7. SUNDAY

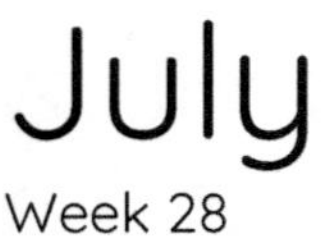

July

Week 28

07/08/19 to 07/14/19

○ 8. MONDAY

DINNER PLANS

○ 9. TUESDAY

○ 10. WEDNESDAY

TO DO

○ 11. THURSDAY

○ 12. FRIDAY

○ 13. SATURDAY / 14. SUNDAY

July

Week 29

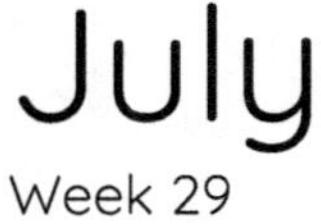

07/15/19 to 07/21/19

O 15. MONDAY

DINNER PLANS

O 16. TUESDAY

O 17. WEDNESDAY

TO DO

O 18. THURSDAY

O 19. FRIDAY

O 20. SATURDAY / 21. SUNDAY

July

Week 30

07/22/19 to 07/28/19

○ 22. MONDAY

DINNER PLANS

○ 23. TUESDAY

○ 24. WEDNESDAY

TO DO

○ 25. THURSDAY

○ 26. FRIDAY

○ 27. SATURDAY / 28. SUNDAY

July

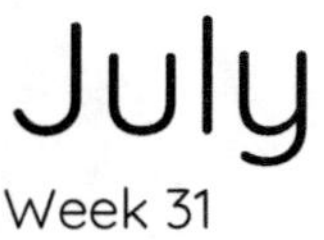

Week 31

07/29/19 to 08/04/19

○ 29. MONDAY

DINNER PLANS

○ 30. TUESDAY

○ 31. WEDNESDAY

TO DO

○ 1. THURSDAY

○ 2. FRIDAY

○ 3. SATURDAY / 4. SUNDAY

August

Week 32

08/05/19 to 08/11/19

○ 5. MONDAY

DINNER PLANS

○ 6. TUESDAY

○ 7. WEDNESDAY

TO DO

○ 8. THURSDAY

○ 9. FRIDAY

○ 10. SATURDAY / 11. SUNDAY

August

Week 33

08/12/19 to 08/18/19

○ 12. MONDAY

DINNER PLANS

○ 13. TUESDAY

○ 14. WEDNESDAY

TO DO

○ 15. THURSDAY

○ 16. FRIDAY

○ 17. SATURDAY / 18. SUNDAY

August

Week 34

08/19/19 to 08/25/19

○ 19. MONDAY

○ 20. TUESDAY

○ 21. WEDNESDAY

○ 22. THURSDAY

○ 23. FRIDAY

○ 24. SATURDAY / 25. SUNDAY

DINNER PLANS

TO DO

August

Week 35

08/26/19 to 09/01/19

O 26. MONDAY

DINNER PLANS

O 27. TUESDAY

O 28. WEDNESDAY

TO DO

O 29. THURSDAY

O 30. FRIDAY

O 31. SATURDAY / 1. SUNDAY

September

Week 36

09/02/19 to 09/08/19

○ 2. MONDAY

DINNER PLANS

○ 3. TUESDAY

○ 4. WEDNESDAY

TO DO

○ 5. THURSDAY

○ 6. FRIDAY

○ 7. SATURDAY / 8. SUNDAY

September

09/09/19 to 09/15/19

○ 9. MONDAY

DINNER PLANS

○ 10. TUESDAY

○ 11. WEDNESDAY

TO DO

○ 12. THURSDAY

○ 13. FRIDAY

○ 14. SATURDAY / 15. SUNDAY

September

Week 38

09/16/19 to 09/22/19

○ 16. MONDAY

DINNER PLANS

○ 17. TUESDAY

○ 18. WEDNESDAY

TO DO

○ 19. THURSDAY

○ 20. FRIDAY

○ 21. SATURDAY / 22. SUNDAY

September

Week 39

09/23/19 to 09/29/19

○ 23. MONDAY

DINNER PLANS

○ 24. TUESDAY

○ 25. WEDNESDAY

TO DO

○ 26. THURSDAY

○ 27. FRIDAY

○ 28. SATURDAY / 29. SUNDAY

September

Week 40

09/30/19 to 10/06/19

○ 30. MONDAY

DINNER PLANS

____

____

____

____

○ 1. TUESDAY

○ 2. WEDNESDAY

TO DO

____

____

○ 3. THURSDAY

____

____

____

○ 4. FRIDAY

____

____

____

____

○ 5. SATURDAY / 6. SUNDAY

____

____

____

October

Week 41

10/07/19 to 10/13/19

○ 7. MONDAY

DINNER PLANS

○ 8. TUESDAY

○ 9. WEDNESDAY

TO DO

○ 10. THURSDAY

○ 11. FRIDAY

○ 12. SATURDAY / 13. SUNDAY

October

10/14/19 to 10/20/19

○ 14. MONDAY

DINNER PLANS

○ 15. TUESDAY

○ 16. WEDNESDAY

TO DO

○ 17. THURSDAY

○ 18. FRIDAY

○ 19. SATURDAY / 20. SUNDAY

October

Week 43

10/21/19 to 10/27/19

◯ 21. MONDAY

DINNER PLANS

◯ 22. TUESDAY

◯ 23. WEDNESDAY

TO DO

◯ 24. THURSDAY

◯ 25. FRIDAY

◯ 26. SATURDAY / 27. SUNDAY

October

Week 44   10/28/19 to 11/03/19

○ 28. MONDAY

DINNER PLANS

○ 29. TUESDAY

○ 30. WEDNESDAY

TO DO

○ 31. THURSDAY

○ 1. FRIDAY

○ 2. SATURDAY / 3. SUNDAY

November

11/04/19 to 11/10/19

○ 4. MONDAY

DINNER PLANS

○ 5. TUESDAY

○ 6. WEDNESDAY

TO DO

○ 7. THURSDAY

○ 8. FRIDAY

○ 9. SATURDAY / 10. SUNDAY

November

Week 46

11/11/19 to 11/17/19

○ 11. MONDAY

DINNER PLANS

○ 12. TUESDAY

○ 13. WEDNESDAY

TO DO

○ 14. THURSDAY

○ 15. FRIDAY

○ 16. SATURDAY / 17. SUNDAY

November

Week 47

11/18/19 to 11/24/19

○ 18. MONDAY

DINNER PLANS

○ 19. TUESDAY

○ 20. WEDNESDAY

TO DO

○ 21. THURSDAY

○ 22. FRIDAY

○ 23. SATURDAY / 24. SUNDAY

November

Week 48

11/25/19 to 12/01/19

○ 25. MONDAY

DINNER PLANS

○ 26. TUESDAY

○ 27. WEDNESDAY

TO DO

○ 28. THURSDAY

○ 29. FRIDAY

○ 30. SATURDAY / 1. SUNDAY

December

Week 49

12/02/19 to 12/08/19

○ 2. MONDAY

DINNER PLANS

○ 3. TUESDAY

○ 4. WEDNESDAY

TO DO

○ 5. THURSDAY

○ 6. FRIDAY

○ 7. SATURDAY / 8. SUNDAY

December

Week 50

12/09/19 to 12/15/19

○ 9. MONDAY

DINNER PLANS

○ 10. TUESDAY

○ 11. WEDNESDAY

TO DO

○ 12. THURSDAY

○ 13. FRIDAY

○ 14. SATURDAY / 15. SUNDAY

December

Week 51

12/16/19 to 12/22/19

○ 16. MONDAY

DINNER PLANS

○ 17. TUESDAY

○ 18. WEDNESDAY

TO DO

○ 19. THURSDAY

○ 20. FRIDAY

○ 21. SATURDAY / 22. SUNDAY

December

Week 52

12/23/19 to 12/29/19

○ 23. MONDAY

DINNER PLANS

○ 24. TUESDAY

○ 25. WEDNESDAY

TO DO

○ 26. THURSDAY

○ 27. FRIDAY

○ 28. SATURDAY / 29. SUNDAY

December

Week 1

12/30/19 to 01/05/20

○ 30. MONDAY

DINNER PLANS

○ 31. TUESDAY

○ 1. WEDNESDAY

TO DO

○ 2. THURSDAY

○ 3. FRIDAY

○ 4. SATURDAY / 5. SUNDAY

Habit Tracker

Month __________

Year __________

Day														
1														
2														
3														
4														
5														
6														
7														
8														
9														
10														
11														
12														
13														
14														
15														
16														
17														
18														
19														
20														
21														
22														
23														
24														
25														
26														
27														
28														
29														
30														
31														

Habit Tracker

Month _______________

Year _______________

Day

1															
2															
3															
4															
5															
6															
7															
8															
9															
10															
11															
12															
13															
14															
15															
16															
17															
18															
19															
20															
21															
22															
23															
24															
25															
26															
27															
28															
29															
30															
31															

Habit Tracker

Month ________________

Year ________________

Day

1													
2													
3													
4													
5													
6													
7													
8													
9													
10													
11													
12													
13													
14													
15													
16													
17													
18													
19													
20													
21													
22													
23													
24													
25													
26													
27													
28													
29													
30													
31													

Habit Tracker

Month __________________

Year __________________

Day															
1															
2															
3															
4															
5															
6															
7															
8															
9															
10															
11															
12															
13															
14															
15															
16															
17															
18															
19															
20															
21															
22															
23															
24															
25															
26															
27															
28															
29															
30															
31															

Habit Tracker

Month ____________________

Year ____________________

Day															
1															
2															
3															
4															
5															
6															
7															
8															
9															
10															
11															
12															
13															
14															
15															
16															
17															
18															
19															
20															
21															
22															
23															
24															
25															
26															
27															
28															
29															
30															
31															

Habit Tracker

Month _______________

Year _______________

Day														
1														
2														
3														
4														
5														
6														
7														
8														
9														
10														
11														
12														
13														
14														
15														
16														
17														
18														
19														
20														
21														
22														
23														
24														
25														
26														
27														
28														
29														
30														
31														

Habit Tracker

Month _______________

Year _______________

Day

1														
2														
3														
4														
5														
6														
7														
8														
9														
10														
11														
12														
13														
14														
15														
16														
17														
18														
19														
20														
21														
22														
23														
24														
25														
26														
27														
28														
29														
30														
31														

Habit Tracker

Month ______________

Year ______________

Day															
1															
2															
3															
4															
5															
6															
7															
8															
9															
10															
11															
12															
13															
14															
15															
16															
17															
18															
19															
20															
21															
22															
23															
24															
25															
26															
27															
28															
29															
30															
31															

Habit Tracker

Month _______________

Year _______________

Day

1														
2														
3														
4														
5														
6														
7														
8														
9														
10														
11														
12														
13														
14														
15														
16														
17														
18														
19														
20														
21														
22														
23														
24														
25														
26														
27														
28														
29														
30														
31														

Habit Tracker

Month _______________

Year _______________

Day

| 1 |
| 2 |
| 3 |
| 4 |
| 5 |
| 6 |
| 7 |
| 8 |
| 9 |
| 10 |
| 11 |
| 12 |
| 13 |
| 14 |
| 15 |
| 16 |
| 17 |
| 18 |
| 19 |
| 20 |
| 21 |
| 22 |
| 23 |
| 24 |
| 25 |
| 26 |
| 27 |
| 28 |
| 29 |
| 30 |
| 31 |

Habit Tracker

Month ________________

Year ________________

Day															
1															
2															
3															
4															
5															
6															
7															
8															
9															
10															
11															
12															
13															
14															
15															
16															
17															
18															
19															
20															
21															
22															
23															
24															
25															
26															
27															
28															
29															
30															
31															

Habit Tracker

Month _______________

Year _______________

Day														
1														
2														
3														
4														
5														
6														
7														
8														
9														
10														
11														
12														
13														
14														
15														
16														
17														
18														
19														
20														
21														
22														
23														
24														
25														
26														
27														
28														
29														
30														
Day 31